CURE TO KIDNEY DISEASE

How to Prevent and Cure Kidney Disease Naturally

DR. ARTHUR MYLES

TABLE OF CONTENTS

INTRODUCTION

The kidneys are remarkable organs that play a vital role in maintaining the body's overall health and well-being. These bean-shaped organs, located on either side of the spine just below the rib cage, are responsible for filtering waste products and excess fluids from the blood, which are then excreted as urine. Beyond waste filtration, the kidneys also help regulate blood pressure, balance electrolytes, and produce hormones that are crucial for red blood cell production and bone health.

Given their multifaceted role, it's no surprise that kidney health is essential for maintaining the body's internal equilibrium, known as homeostasis. When the kidneys are functioning properly, they keep the body in a state of balance, but when they are compromised, the effects can be far-reaching and severe.

In recent years, there has been a growing interest in natural and holistic approaches to health, including kidney care. Many people are seeking ways to prevent kidney disease or manage existing conditions through diet, lifestyle changes, and herbal remedies. This shift towards natural methods is driven by a desire to reduce dependence on pharmaceutical treatments, which can come with side effects, and to take a proactive role in maintaining health.

Natural approaches to kidney health focus on prevention, emphasizing the importance of hydration, a balanced diet, regular exercise, and stress management. These strategies not only support kidney function but also enhance overall health, helping to prevent conditions that can lead to kidney damage, such as high blood pressure and diabetes.

For those already dealing with kidney issues, natural remedies can complement conventional treatments. Herbal supplements, dietary adjustments, and lifestyle changes can help manage symptoms, slow the progression of kidney disease, and improve quality of life. However, it is crucial to approach these methods with caution and to work in conjunction with healthcare professionals to ensure safety and effectiveness.

This guide is designed to provide a comprehensive overview of natural ways to support kidney health, offering both preventative strategies and management techniques for those with kidney disease. You will find practical advice on how to incorporate kidney-friendly foods into your diet, tips for staying hydrated, and guidance on using herbal remedies safely. The guide also addresses the importance of monitoring kidney function and knowing when to seek medical advice.

Whether you are looking to maintain healthy kidneys or seeking natural ways to manage kidney disease, this guide aims to empower you with the knowledge and tools to take control of your kidney health. By adopting the strategies outlined in this guide, you can take proactive steps towards preventing kidney disease or managing it more effectively, all while embracing a more natural and holistic approach to your well-being.

CHAPTER 1
Kidney Function and Common Kidney Diseases

Kidney Function

The kidneys are essential organs with a complex and critical role in maintaining the body's internal environment. Each kidney is about the size of a fist and contains around a million tiny filtering units called nephrons. These nephrons are responsible for the kidneys' primary functions:

Filtration of Blood: The kidneys filter about 120 to 150 quarts of blood daily to remove waste products and excess fluids. This filtration process occurs in the nephrons, where blood is passed through tiny capillaries and filtered through a structure called the glomerulus. The filtered fluid then passes through a series of tubules, where essential substances like glucose, sodium, and water are reabsorbed back into the blood, while waste products are excreted as urine.

Regulation of Electrolytes and Fluids: The kidneys regulate the balance of electrolytes, such as sodium, potassium, and calcium, which are crucial for nerve function, muscle contraction, and maintaining the body's acid-base balance. They also control the volume of fluids in the body, ensuring that blood pressure remains within a healthy range.

Hormone Production

Erythropoietin (EPO): The kidneys produce EPO, a hormone that stimulates the bone marrow to produce red blood cells. This process is crucial for preventing anemia.

Renin: The kidneys secrete renin, an enzyme that regulates blood pressure by controlling the constriction of blood vessels and the balance of sodium and water in the body.

Calcitriol: The active form of vitamin D, calcitriol, is also produced by the kidneys. This hormone helps maintain healthy bones by regulating calcium and phosphate levels in the blood.

Detoxification: The kidneys play a key role in detoxifying the body by filtering out harmful substances, such as metabolic waste, drugs, and toxins, which are then excreted in the urine.

Common Kidney Diseases

Kidney diseases occur when the kidneys become damaged and are unable to perform their vital functions effectively. These conditions can range from acute, short-term issues to chronic, long-lasting diseases that can lead to kidney failure. Understanding the common kidney diseases and their causes is essential for prevention and early intervention.

Chronic Kidney Disease (CKD)
CKD is a long-term condition characterized by gradual loss of kidney function over time. It is often a result of underlying conditions like high blood pressure and diabetes.
Causes: Hypertension, diabetes, glomerulonephritis (inflammation of the kidney's filtering units), and polycystic kidney disease are common causes.

Symptoms: Early stages may be asymptomatic, but as the disease progresses, symptoms such as fatigue, swelling (edema), changes in urination, and high blood pressure may occur.
Complications: CKD can lead to complications such as anemia, cardiovascular disease, and bone disease. If untreated, it can progress to end-stage renal disease (ESRD), requiring dialysis or a kidney transplant.

Acute Kidney Injury (AKI)
AKI is a sudden decline in kidney function, often occurring within hours or days. It is typically a response to a severe illness, injury, or certain medications.
Causes: Severe infections, dehydration, trauma, and exposure to nephrotoxic drugs can cause AKI.
Symptoms: Rapid onset of symptoms such as decreased urine output, swelling, nausea, and confusion. AKI can be reversible if treated promptly.
Complications: If untreated, AKI can lead to chronic kidney disease or permanent kidney damage.

Glomerulonephritis

Glomerulonephritis is inflammation of the glomeruli, the tiny filtering units within the kidneys. It can be acute or chronic.

Causes: Infections (like streptococcal infections), autoimmune diseases (such as lupus), and certain drugs can trigger glomerulonephritis.

Symptoms: Blood in the urine (hematuria), protein in the urine (proteinuria), high blood pressure, and swelling in the hands and feet.

Complications: Chronic glomerulonephritis can lead to kidney failure over time if not managed properly.

Polycystic Kidney Disease (PKD)

PKD is a genetic disorder characterized by the growth of numerous cysts in the kidneys. These cysts can enlarge the kidneys and interfere with their function.

Causes: PKD is usually inherited in an autosomal dominant pattern, meaning a person needs only one copy of the defective gene to develop the condition.

Symptoms: High blood pressure, back or side pain, headaches, and blood in the urine. Over time, PKD can lead to kidney failure.

Complications: PKD can cause chronic kidney disease, liver cysts, and aneurysms in the brain.

Kidney Stones
Kidney stones are hard deposits of minerals and salts that form inside the kidneys. They can cause significant pain when they pass through the urinary tract.

Causes: Dehydration, high levels of calcium or oxalate in the urine, and certain dietary factors can contribute to kidney stone formation.

Symptoms: Severe pain in the side and back, pain during urination, and blood in the urine. Nausea and vomiting may also occur.

Complications: Large stones can obstruct the urinary tract, leading to infections or kidney damage. In severe cases, surgery may be required to remove the stones.

Urinary Tract Infections (UTIs)
UTIs are infections that affect the urinary system, including the kidneys. When the infection reaches the kidneys, it is known as pyelonephritis, a serious condition that requires prompt treatment.

Causes: Bacteria, typically E. coli, are the most common cause of UTIs. Poor hygiene, sexual activity, and blockages in the urinary tract can increase the risk.

Symptoms: Frequent urination, pain or burning during urination, cloudy or strong-smelling urine, and pelvic pain. If the infection reaches the kidneys, symptoms may include fever, chills, and back pain.

Complications: Recurrent UTIs can lead to kidney damage, especially if the infection spreads to the kidneys.

Understanding kidney function and the common diseases that can affect these vital organs is the first step towards prevention and early intervention. By recognizing the signs and symptoms of kidney disease, you can take proactive measures to protect your kidney health and seek medical attention when necessary. This knowledge forms the foundation for the natural approaches discussed in the subsequent chapters, helping you to maintain healthy kidneys and prevent or manage kidney disease naturally.

CHAPTER 2
Prevention Strategies

Preventing kidney disease is crucial for maintaining overall health and well-being. By adopting a proactive approach, you can significantly reduce the risk of kidney-related issues. This chapter outlines essential strategies for preventing kidney disease, focusing on hydration, diet, lifestyle choices, and natural remedies.

Staying Hydrated

Hydration is one of the most important factors in kidney health. Proper hydration helps the kidneys effectively filter waste and toxins from the blood, preventing the formation of kidney stones and other issues.

Daily Water Intake: Aim to drink at least 8-10 glasses of water per day. Your specific needs may vary depending on factors such as climate, physical activity, and overall health. Adjust your intake based on your body's signals, like thirst and urine color—pale yellow is a sign of good hydration.

Avoid Sugary Drinks: Soft drinks, energy drinks, and other sugary beverages can increase the risk of kidney stones and other kidney-related issues. Opt for water, herbal teas, or infused water with lemon or cucumber instead.

Healthy Diet for Kidney Health

A balanced diet plays a key role in maintaining kidney health. The following dietary guidelines can help support your kidneys and prevent disease:

Reduce Sodium Intake: Excessive sodium can increase blood pressure, leading to kidney damage over time. Limit processed foods, fast foods, and canned goods, as these are often high in sodium. Instead, use herbs and spices to flavor your meals.

Choose Kidney-Friendly Foods:

Fruits and Vegetables: Incorporate antioxidant-rich fruits and vegetables, such as berries, apples, bell peppers, and leafy greens. These foods help protect the kidneys from oxidative stress and inflammation.

Whole Grains: Whole grains like brown rice, quinoa, and oats provide essential nutrients without burdening the kidneys.

Lean Proteins: Opt for moderate portions of lean proteins, such as fish, chicken, tofu, and legumes. While protein is important, too much can strain the kidneys.

Control Potassium and Phosphorus Levels: While potassium and phosphorus are essential minerals, excessive amounts can be harmful to those with existing kidney conditions. Foods high in potassium include bananas, oranges, potatoes, and tomatoes, while high-phosphorus foods include dairy, nuts, and certain whole grains. If you are at risk for kidney disease, consult with a healthcare professional to determine the right levels for your diet.

Managing Blood Pressure and Blood Sugar
High blood pressure and diabetes are two of the leading causes of kidney disease. By managing these conditions, you can protect your kidneys from damage.

Blood Pressure Control: Maintain a healthy blood pressure level (typically below 120/80 mm Hg). Regular physical activity, a low-sodium diet, and stress management techniques like meditation or deep breathing exercises can help keep your blood pressure in check.
Blood Sugar Management: If you have diabetes or are at risk, monitor your blood sugar levels regularly. A diet rich in fiber, low in refined sugars, and balanced in carbohydrates can help maintain stable blood sugar levels. Regular exercise also plays a crucial role in blood sugar management.

Limiting Alcohol and Avoiding Smoking
Alcohol and smoking can have detrimental effects on kidney health. By reducing or eliminating these substances, you can protect your kidneys and improve overall health.

Limit Alcohol Consumption: Excessive alcohol intake can lead to dehydration, high blood pressure, and liver damage, all of which can negatively impact the kidneys. If you drink alcohol, do so in moderation— no more than one drink per day for women and two drinks per day for men.

Quit Smoking: Smoking increases the risk of kidney disease by reducing blood flow to the kidneys and causing damage to kidney tissues. It also exacerbates high blood pressure and diabetes, which are major risk factors for kidney disease. Quitting smoking is one of the best steps you can take to protect your kidneys.

Herbal Support for Prevention

Certain herbs have been traditionally used to support kidney health and prevent disease. Incorporating these into your routine can provide additional protection for your kidneys:

Dandelion Root: Known for its diuretic properties, dandelion root helps increase urine production, aiding in the removal of toxins and excess fluids from the body. It can be consumed as a tea or taken in supplement form.

Nettle Leaf: Nettle leaf is rich in antioxidants and has anti-inflammatory properties, which can help protect the kidneys from damage. It also supports overall urinary tract health. Nettle leaf tea is a popular way to consume this herb.

Cranberry: Cranberry is effective in preventing urinary tract infections (UTIs), which can lead to kidney infections if left untreated. Regular consumption of unsweetened cranberry juice or cranberry supplements can help maintain urinary tract health and reduce the risk of infection-related kidney damage.

Regular Physical Activity

Exercise is essential for overall health and plays a significant role in preventing kidney disease. Regular physical activity helps maintain healthy blood pressure, blood sugar levels, and body weight, all of which are critical for kidney health.

Exercise Recommendations: Aim for at least 150 minutes of moderate-intensity exercise per week, such as brisk walking, cycling, or swimming. Incorporate strength training exercises at least twice a week to improve muscle strength and metabolic health.

Staying Active: In addition to structured exercise, stay active throughout the day by taking breaks to walk, stretch, or engage in light physical activity. This helps improve circulation and supports kidney function.

Stress Management

Chronic stress can contribute to high blood pressure and other health issues that negatively impact the kidneys. Managing stress is an important aspect of kidney disease prevention.

Mindfulness and Meditation: Practices like mindfulness meditation can help reduce stress and promote relaxation. Even a few minutes of deep breathing or quiet reflection each day can have a positive impact on your overall well-being.

Yoga and Tai Chi: These gentle forms of exercise combine physical movement with deep breathing and meditation, making them effective for both stress reduction and physical fitness.
Adequate Sleep: Getting enough sleep is crucial for stress management and overall health. Aim for 7-9 hours of quality sleep each night to support your body's natural repair processes and maintain kidney health.

Preventing kidney disease requires a holistic approach that combines hydration, a balanced diet, regular exercise, and stress management. By adopting these prevention strategies, you can support your kidneys' health, reduce the risk of developing kidney disease, and enhance your overall well-being. These proactive measures not only protect your kidneys but also promote a healthier lifestyle, ensuring that your body remains in optimal condition.

CHAPTER 3
Kidney-Friendly Diet

A kidney-friendly diet is crucial for maintaining kidney health and preventing or managing kidney disease. This chapter will guide you through the essential dietary components, foods to include, and those to limit or avoid, ensuring that your kidneys function optimally.

Foods to Include: Antioxidant-Rich Choices

Antioxidants play a vital role in protecting the kidneys from oxidative stress and inflammation, which can lead to kidney damage. Incorporating a variety of antioxidant-rich foods into your diet can help support kidney function and overall health.

Berries: Blueberries, strawberries, raspberries, and blackberries are packed with antioxidants, vitamins, and fiber. These fruits are excellent choices for a kidney-friendly diet.

Apples: Apples are high in fiber and low in potassium, making them ideal for kidney health. They help reduce cholesterol, inflammation, and blood sugar levels.

Red Bell Peppers: These peppers are low in potassium and high in vitamins A, C, and B6. They also contain lycopene, an antioxidant that helps protect against certain cancers.

Cabbage: Cabbage is a low-potassium vegetable rich in vitamins K, C, and B6, as well as fiber. It's a versatile addition to salads, soups, and stir-fries.

Cauliflower: Cauliflower is another low-potassium vegetable that's high in vitamin C, fiber, and folate. It can be used as a substitute for higher-potassium foods like potatoes.

Controlling Protein Intake
While protein is essential for the body, too much can strain the kidneys, especially if kidney function is already compromised. Balancing protein intake is crucial for maintaining kidney health.

Lean Proteins: Choose lean sources of protein such as chicken, turkey, fish, and plant-based options like tofu and legumes. These proteins are easier on the kidneys compared to red meat.

Portion Control: Focus on moderate portions of protein-rich foods. A typical serving size is about the size of the palm of your hand or 3-4 ounces per meal.

Plant-Based Proteins: Incorporate more plant-based proteins like beans, lentils, and quinoa into your diet. These options are lower in saturated fats and can be easier for the kidneys to process.

Limiting Sodium, Potassium, and Phosphorus

Excessive intake of sodium, potassium, and phosphorus can be harmful to the kidneys, especially for individuals with kidney disease. Monitoring and controlling these minerals in your diet is important for kidney health.

Sodium:

Limit Processed Foods: Processed and pre-packaged foods are often high in sodium. Opt for fresh or minimally processed options whenever possible.

Use Herbs and Spices: Instead of salt, flavor your meals with herbs, spices, lemon juice, or vinegar. Fresh garlic, rosemary, basil, and thyme are great choices.

Read Labels: Check food labels for sodium content, and choose low-sodium or no-salt-added products.

Potassium:

Monitor Potassium Intake: High potassium levels can be dangerous for those with kidney issues. Limit high-potassium foods like bananas, oranges, potatoes, tomatoes, and spinach if advised by your healthcare provider.

Choose Low-Potassium Alternatives: Opt for apples, berries, carrots, cucumbers, and lettuce, which are lower in potassium.

Cooking Tips: Leaching vegetables by soaking them in water before cooking can help reduce their potassium content.

Phosphorus:
Avoid High-Phosphorus Foods: Limit dairy products, nuts, seeds, whole grains, and certain fish that are high in phosphorus. Processed foods and sodas often contain added phosphorus, so read labels carefully.

Choose Phosphorus Binders: For those with advanced kidney disease, phosphorus binders prescribed by a doctor can help control phosphorus levels.

Benefits of Omega-3 Fatty Acids
Omega-3 fatty acids are essential fats that have anti-inflammatory properties and are beneficial for heart and kidney health. Incorporating omega-3s into your diet can help reduce inflammation and lower the risk of kidney disease progression.

Fatty Fish: Salmon, mackerel, sardines, and trout are excellent sources of omega-3 fatty acids. Aim to include these fish in your diet at least twice a week.

Flaxseeds and Chia Seeds: These plant-based sources of omega-3s can be easily added to smoothies, oatmeal, or yogurt. They also provide additional fiber, which supports digestive health.

Walnuts: Walnuts are another plant-based source of omega-3s. A small handful as a snack or added to salads can boost your intake of these healthy fats.

Hydration: The Importance of Fluids
Proper hydration is vital for kidney function, as it helps the kidneys filter waste and toxins from the blood. However, the amount of fluid intake may need to be adjusted based on your kidney function and medical advice.

Water: Water is the best choice for hydration. Aim to drink 8-10 glasses of water per day, or as advised by your healthcare provider. If you have kidney disease, your doctor may recommend a specific fluid intake.

Herbal Teas: Herbal teas like chamomile, peppermint, and dandelion root can be hydrating and offer additional health benefits. Avoid teas with high levels of caffeine, as they can lead to dehydration.

Limit Sugary and Carbonated Beverages: These drinks can contribute to kidney stones and other kidney problems. Opt for water or herbal teas instead.

Meal Planning Tips for a Kidney-Friendly Diet
Planning your meals with kidney health in mind can help you stay on track and ensure that you are getting the right nutrients while avoiding harmful foods.

Balanced Plates: Fill half your plate with fruits and vegetables, a quarter with lean proteins, and the remaining quarter with whole grains. This balance supports kidney health and overall nutrition.

Meal Prep: Preparing meals in advance can help you stick to a kidney-friendly diet, avoid processed foods, and control portion sizes. Cook large batches of kidney-friendly foods and store them in portion-sized containers for easy access during the week.

Consult a Dietitian: If you have kidney disease or are at risk, working with a registered dietitian can help you create a personalized meal plan that meets your nutritional needs while protecting your kidneys.

A kidney-friendly diet is essential for maintaining kidney function and preventing kidney disease. By incorporating antioxidant-rich foods, controlling protein intake, and managing sodium, potassium, and phosphorus levels, you can support your kidney health. Additionally, including omega-3 fatty acids, staying hydrated, and planning balanced meals are key strategies for promoting overall well-being and protecting your kidneys from damage. Making these dietary changes can have a profound impact on your health, helping you lead a healthier, more vibrant life.

CHAPTER 4

Lifestyle Changes for Kidney Health

Making positive lifestyle changes is essential for maintaining kidney health and preventing kidney disease. This chapter explores various lifestyle adjustments that can significantly impact kidney function, reduce the risk of kidney disease, and promote overall well-being.

Regular Physical Activity

Exercise plays a crucial role in maintaining healthy kidneys by helping to regulate blood pressure, control blood sugar levels, and manage body weight.

Cardiovascular Exercise: Engage in aerobic activities like brisk walking, cycling, swimming, or dancing for at least 150 minutes per week. These exercises help improve circulation, lower blood pressure, and enhance overall cardiovascular health, which directly benefits the kidneys.

Strength Training: Incorporate strength training exercises, such as weight lifting or bodyweight exercises, at least twice a week. Building muscle mass can help improve metabolism and support healthy blood sugar levels, reducing the strain on your kidneys.

Consistency: The key to reaping the benefits of exercise is consistency. Find activities you enjoy and make them a regular part of your routine. Even short bursts of physical activity throughout the day can add up to significant health benefits.

Maintaining a Healthy Weight

Excess weight can increase the risk of developing conditions like high blood pressure and diabetes, which are leading causes of kidney disease. Achieving and maintaining a healthy weight is important for kidney health.

Balanced Diet: Follow a kidney-friendly diet that emphasizes whole foods, fruits, vegetables, lean proteins, and healthy fats. Avoid processed foods, sugary snacks, and high-calorie beverages.

Portion Control: Be mindful of portion sizes, especially when it comes to high-calorie foods. Eating smaller, balanced meals throughout the day can help you maintain a healthy weight.

Mindful Eating: Practice mindful eating by paying attention to hunger and fullness cues, eating slowly, and savoring your food. This can help prevent overeating and support weight management.

Managing Stress

Chronic stress can negatively impact kidney health by contributing to high blood pressure and other health issues. Learning to manage stress effectively is essential for protecting your kidneys.

Mindfulness and Meditation: Engage in mindfulness practices, such as meditation or deep breathing exercises, to reduce stress and promote relaxation. Even a few minutes of quiet reflection each day can have a calming effect on the mind and body.

Yoga and Tai Chi: These gentle forms of exercise combine physical movement with breath control and meditation, making them effective for both stress reduction and physical health. Regular practice can help lower blood pressure and improve overall well-being.

Time Management: Organize your daily tasks and set realistic goals to reduce feelings of overwhelm. Prioritize self-care and make time for activities that bring you joy and relaxation.

Avoiding Harmful Substances
Certain substances can have a detrimental effect on kidney health. By avoiding or limiting these substances, you can protect your kidneys and improve your overall health.

Tobacco: Smoking reduces blood flow to the kidneys, damages kidney tissue, and increases the risk of kidney disease. Quitting smoking is one of the best things you can do for your kidney health. Seek support through cessation programs, counseling, or nicotine replacement therapies if needed.

Alcohol: Excessive alcohol consumption can lead to dehydration, high blood pressure, and liver damage, all of which can negatively impact the kidneys. Limit alcohol intake to no more than one drink per day for women and two drinks per day for men, or avoid it altogether.

Over-the-Counter Medications: Certain over-the-counter medications, such as nonsteroidal anti-inflammatory drugs (NSAIDs) like ibuprofen, can cause kidney damage if used excessively or for long periods. Always follow the recommended dosage, and consult with your healthcare provider before taking any new medications.

Sleep and Kidney Health

Adequate sleep is vital for overall health, including kidney function. Poor sleep patterns can lead to high blood pressure and other health problems that strain the kidneys.

Sleep Hygiene: Establish a regular sleep routine by going to bed and waking up at the same time each day, even on weekends. Create a calming bedtime ritual, such as reading, listening to soothing music, or practicing relaxation techniques.

Comfortable Sleep Environment: Ensure that your bedroom is conducive to sleep by keeping it cool, dark, and quiet. Invest in a comfortable mattress and pillows to support restful sleep.

Limit Stimulants: Avoid caffeine and heavy meals close to bedtime, as they can interfere with sleep. Also, limit screen time before bed, as the blue light emitted by phones and computers can disrupt your sleep cycle.

Regular Health Check-Ups

Routine health check-ups are important for monitoring kidney function and catching any potential issues early. Regular visits to your healthcare provider can help you stay on top of your kidney health.

Blood Pressure Monitoring: Keep track of your blood pressure, as high blood pressure is a major risk factor for kidney disease. Regular monitoring and management are crucial for kidney health.

Blood Sugar Control: If you have diabetes or are at risk, regularly monitor your blood sugar levels to prevent damage to the kidneys. Work with your healthcare provider to manage your condition effectively.

Kidney Function Tests: Ask your doctor about getting regular kidney function tests, such as blood urea nitrogen (BUN) and creatinine levels, especially if you have risk factors for kidney disease.

Hydration and Kidney Health

Proper hydration is essential for kidney function, as it helps flush out toxins and prevent kidney stones.

Drink Water: Water is the best beverage for hydration. Aim to drink 8-10 glasses of water per day, or more if you are physically active or live in a hot climate. Listen to your body's thirst signals to guide your fluid intake.

Limit Sugary Drinks: Sugary beverages like sodas and energy drinks can increase the risk of kidney stones and other kidney-related issues. Opt for water, herbal teas, or infused water with natural flavors like lemon or cucumber.

Monitor Fluid Intake: If you have a condition that requires you to limit fluid intake, such as advanced kidney disease, follow your healthcare provider's recommendations to avoid overloading your kidneys.

Lifestyle changes play a crucial role in maintaining kidney health and preventing kidney disease. By incorporating regular physical activity, maintaining a healthy weight, managing stress, avoiding harmful substances, getting adequate sleep, and staying hydrated, you can support your kidneys and improve your overall health. Regular health check-ups and monitoring are also essential for catching any potential issues early and ensuring that your kidneys remain healthy and functional. These lifestyle adjustments not only protect your kidneys but also contribute to a healthier, more fulfilling life.

CHAPTER 5

Natural Remedies for Managing Kidney Disease

While conventional treatments are often necessary for managing kidney disease, natural remedies can complement these treatments and help support kidney function. This chapter explores various natural remedies that may aid in managing kidney disease, reduce symptoms, and promote overall kidney health.

Herbal Remedies

Certain herbs have been traditionally used to support kidney health and manage symptoms of kidney disease. Incorporating these herbs into your routine can provide additional benefits.

Dandelion Root: Dandelion root acts as a natural diuretic, increasing urine production and helping to flush out toxins. It can be consumed as a tea or taken in supplement form. Dandelion is also rich in vitamins A and C, which support kidney function.

Nettle Leaf: Nettle leaf is known for its anti-inflammatory properties and ability to support urinary tract health. It can be consumed as a tea or used in cooking. Nettle leaf is also a good source of iron, which is beneficial for those with anemia related to kidney disease.

Astragalus: Astragalus is an adaptogenic herb that helps protect the kidneys from damage by reducing inflammation and oxidative stress. It can also improve immune function, making it helpful for those with chronic kidney disease. Astragalus is typically taken in capsule or tincture form.

Corn Silk: Corn silk has diuretic properties and can help reduce water retention, which is often an issue for those with kidney disease. It also soothes the urinary tract and may help prevent infections. Corn silk can be brewed into a tea.

Dietary Supplements
In addition to a kidney-friendly diet, certain supplements can provide essential nutrients that support kidney health. Always consult with a healthcare provider before starting any new supplements, especially if you have kidney disease.

Omega-3 Fatty Acids: Omega-3s help reduce inflammation and lower the risk of kidney disease progression. Fish oil supplements are a common source of omega-3s, but they can also be obtained from flaxseed oil or algae-based supplements for those who prefer plant-based options.

Coenzyme Q10 (CoQ10): CoQ10 is an antioxidant that helps protect the kidneys from oxidative damage. It also supports heart health, which is closely linked to kidney function. CoQ10 supplements may help improve kidney function in those with chronic kidney disease.

Vitamin D: Vitamin D is essential for bone health and immune function. Since kidney disease can impair the body's ability to activate vitamin D, supplementation may be necessary. Vitamin D3 is the preferred form for supplementation.

Probiotics: Probiotics support gut health, which in turn can influence kidney health. Certain probiotic strains may help reduce uremic toxins, which accumulate in the blood due to impaired kidney function. Probiotics can be taken as supplements or consumed through fermented foods like yogurt, kefir, and sauerkraut.

Detoxifying Foods and Drinks
Incorporating detoxifying foods and drinks into your diet can help support kidney function by promoting the elimination of toxins and reducing the burden on the kidneys.

Cranberry Juice: Unsweetened cranberry juice is known for its ability to prevent urinary tract infections (UTIs), which can lead to kidney infections if left untreated. Regular consumption of cranberry juice can help maintain urinary tract health.

Parsley: Parsley has natural diuretic properties, helping to increase urine production and flush out excess fluids and toxins. It can be added to salads, smoothies, or used as a garnish in various dishes.

Watermelon: Watermelon is hydrating and has a high water content, which helps promote urine production and detoxification. It is also low in potassium, making it a good choice for those with kidney disease who need to monitor their potassium intake.

Cucumber: Cucumber is another hydrating food that supports kidney function. It is low in calories and provides a refreshing, kidney-friendly snack. Cucumbers can also be added to salads or infused in water for a detoxifying drink.

Acupuncture and Traditional Chinese Medicine (TCM)

Acupuncture and Traditional Chinese Medicine (TCM) offer holistic approaches to managing kidney disease by addressing the body's energy flow and promoting balance.

Acupuncture: Acupuncture involves the insertion of thin needles into specific points on the body to stimulate energy flow (Qi) and improve organ function. It can help reduce symptoms like pain, fatigue, and fluid retention associated with kidney disease.

TCM Herbal Formulas: TCM practitioners often prescribe herbal formulas tailored to an individual's specific condition. These formulas may include a combination of herbs like Rehmannia, Cornus, and Poria, which are believed to support kidney health and overall vitality.

Mind-Body Techniques

Mind-body techniques can help manage stress and improve overall well-being, which is important for those dealing with chronic kidney disease.

Meditation and Mindfulness: Meditation and mindfulness practices can help reduce stress, lower blood pressure, and improve emotional well-being. These practices involve focusing on the present moment, breathing deeply, and letting go of stressors.

Yoga: Yoga combines physical movement with breath control and meditation, making it an effective practice for managing stress and promoting relaxation. Certain yoga poses can also help improve circulation and support kidney function.

Guided Imagery: Guided imagery involves visualizing positive, healing images in the mind, which can promote relaxation and reduce anxiety. It is a helpful technique for managing the emotional and psychological aspects of chronic kidney disease.

Aromatherapy

Aromatherapy uses essential oils to promote relaxation and alleviate symptoms associated with kidney disease.

Lavender Oil: Lavender oil is known for its calming effects and can help reduce stress and anxiety. It can be diffused in the air, added to a bath, or applied topically (diluted with a carrier oil) for a soothing massage.

Peppermint Oil: Peppermint oil has a refreshing scent that can help relieve nausea, a common symptom in those with kidney disease. It can be inhaled directly from the bottle, diffused, or applied topically (diluted) to the temples.

Eucalyptus Oil: Eucalyptus oil can help improve respiratory function and provide relief from congestion, which can be beneficial for those with kidney-related fluid retention. It can be diffused or inhaled through steam inhalation.

Natural remedies can play a supportive role in managing kidney disease, complementing conventional treatments and promoting overall kidney health. Herbal remedies, dietary supplements, detoxifying foods, acupuncture, mind-body techniques, and aromatherapy all offer potential benefits for those dealing with kidney disease. However, it's important to consult with a healthcare provider before starting any new natural remedy, especially if you have existing kidney conditions or are taking medications. By integrating these natural approaches into your routine, you can take a proactive role in managing your kidney health and enhancing your quality of life.

CHAPTER 6

Case Studies and Success Stories

Real-life experiences can provide valuable insights and inspiration for those managing kidney disease. This chapter presents case studies and success stories of individuals who have successfully improved their kidney health through natural remedies, lifestyle changes, and holistic approaches.

Case Study 1: Reversing Early-Stage Kidney Disease Through Diet and Lifestyle

Background: John, a 52-year-old man, was diagnosed with early-stage chronic kidney disease (CKD) during a routine health check-up. His condition was primarily attributed to long-standing hypertension and a poor diet high in sodium and processed foods. John was advised to make significant lifestyle changes to prevent the progression of his kidney disease.

Approach:

Dietary Changes: John worked with a registered dietitian to adopt a kidney-friendly diet, focusing on low-sodium, low-protein, and antioxidant-rich foods. He incorporated more fresh fruits, vegetables, and lean proteins while avoiding processed and high-potassium foods.

Exercise Routine: John started a regular exercise regimen, including 30 minutes of brisk walking five days a week. This helped him manage his blood pressure and improve cardiovascular health.

Herbal Supplements: After consulting with his healthcare provider, John began taking omega-3 fatty acid supplements to reduce inflammation and support kidney function.

Outcome:

Over the course of a year, John's kidney function improved significantly, as reflected in his blood test results. His eGFR (estimated glomerular filtration rate) stabilized, and he successfully managed his blood pressure without the need for additional medications. John's proactive approach to diet and lifestyle changes played a critical role in halting the progression of his kidney disease.

Case Study 2: Managing Kidney Disease with Holistic Therapies

Background: Maria, a 60-year-old woman, was diagnosed with stage 3 CKD. In addition to conventional treatments, Maria sought holistic therapies to help manage her condition. She was particularly interested in reducing her reliance on medication and improving her overall well-being.

Approach:

Acupuncture: Maria began receiving weekly acupuncture treatments to help manage symptoms such as fatigue, swelling, and high blood pressure.

These sessions also aimed to balance her body's energy flow and support kidney health.

Traditional Chinese Medicine (TCM): Maria's TCM practitioner prescribed an herbal formula specifically designed to support kidney function and overall vitality. This formula included herbs like Rehmannia and Cornus.

Mind-Body Practices: Maria incorporated yoga and meditation into her daily routine to manage stress and promote relaxation. These practices helped her maintain emotional balance and improve her quality of life.

Outcome:
Maria experienced a reduction in symptoms, such as decreased swelling and improved energy levels. Her blood pressure was better controlled, and she felt more balanced and at peace. While her kidney function remained stable, the combination of holistic therapies and conventional treatments helped her manage her condition more effectively and improved her overall well-being.

Case Study 3: Overcoming Kidney Stones with Natural Remedies
Background: David, a 45-year-old man, had a history of recurrent kidney stones. He was looking for natural ways to prevent future stones and avoid the pain and complications associated with them.

Approach:
Hydration: David increased his water intake to ensure he stayed well-hydrated, aiming for at least 10 glasses of water per day. He also drank herbal teas like dandelion root and corn silk to support kidney function and promote detoxification.

Dietary Modifications: David reduced his intake of oxalate-rich foods like spinach, nuts, and chocolate, which are known to contribute to the formation of kidney stones. He also avoided high-sodium foods to reduce the risk of stone formation.
Natural Supplements: Under the guidance of a healthcare professional, David started taking magnesium and potassium citrate supplements, both of which are known to reduce the risk of stone formation.

Outcome:
David successfully prevented the recurrence of kidney stones by adhering to his new hydration and dietary regimen. Over the next two years, he did not experience any new stone formations, and he reported feeling healthier and more energetic overall. His commitment to natural remedies and preventive measures allowed him to avoid further kidney stone episodes.

Success Story: Healing from CKD with a Plant-Based Diet

Background: Sarah, a 48-year-old woman, was diagnosed with stage 2 CKD. Concerned about the potential progression of her condition, she decided to adopt a plant-based diet as part of her treatment plan.

Approach:

Plant-Based Diet: Sarah transitioned to a plant-based diet, focusing on whole foods such as fruits, vegetables, legumes, and whole grains. She eliminated animal products, processed foods, and refined sugars from her diet.

Detoxifying Foods: Sarah included detoxifying foods like parsley, watermelon, and cucumber in her meals to support kidney function and promote natural detoxification.

Regular Check-Ups: Sarah continued to see her healthcare provider regularly to monitor her kidney function and make any necessary adjustments to her treatment plan.

Outcome:

After six months on a plant-based diet, Sarah's kidney function improved, and her eGFR levels increased, indicating better kidney performance. She also experienced weight loss, improved energy levels, and better overall health. Sarah's success with a plant-based diet highlights the potential benefits of dietary changes in managing kidney disease.

Case Study: Reducing Dialysis Frequency with Natural Support

Background: Paul, a 65-year-old man, was on dialysis due to advanced CKD. He was determined to explore natural ways to support his kidney function and reduce his reliance on dialysis.

Approach:

Herbal Support: Paul began using nettle leaf and astragalus supplements, which he discussed with his nephrologist, to support his remaining kidney function and reduce inflammation.

Hydration Management: Paul carefully managed his fluid intake, balancing the need to stay hydrated with the restrictions required for his dialysis regimen.

Acupuncture: Paul added acupuncture to his treatment plan, focusing on improving circulation, reducing fluid retention, and enhancing overall kidney function.

Outcome:

Paul experienced a reduction in symptoms such as fatigue and fluid retention. Over time, his nephrologist noted a slight improvement in his kidney function, allowing him to reduce the frequency of his dialysis sessions. While he remained on dialysis, the natural support helped improve his quality of life and gave him more energy and vitality.

These case studies and success stories demonstrate the potential benefits of integrating natural remedies, lifestyle changes, and holistic therapies into the management of kidney disease. While each individual's journey is unique, the common thread is the proactive approach to kidney health, combining conventional treatments with natural support. These stories serve as inspiration and offer hope to others facing similar challenges, showing that positive changes and a commitment to health can lead to significant improvements in kidney function and overall well-being.

CHAPTER 7
When to Seek Medical Attention

While natural remedies and lifestyle changes can be beneficial for managing kidney health, there are situations where medical attention is essential. Recognizing when to seek medical care is crucial for preventing complications and ensuring proper management of kidney disease. This chapter outlines key indicators that warrant professional medical evaluation.

Persistent Symptoms

Certain symptoms can signal worsening kidney function or complications. If you experience any of the following symptoms persistently, seek medical attention:

Severe Fatigue: Chronic fatigue or feeling excessively tired despite adequate rest can indicate worsening kidney function or anemia, a common complication of kidney disease.

Swelling: Swelling in the legs, ankles, or face that does not improve with dietary changes or natural remedies may be a sign of fluid retention or worsening kidney function.

Shortness of Breath: Difficulty breathing or shortness of breath can be a sign of fluid buildup in the lungs, which may be related to kidney issues.

Changes in Urine Output

Changes in urine output can indicate problems with kidney function. Seek medical advice if you notice:

Decreased Urine Output: Significant reduction in urine production or completely stopped urination can be a sign of acute kidney injury or severe kidney dysfunction.

Blood in Urine: The presence of blood in the urine (hematuria) can indicate kidney stones, infections, or other serious conditions requiring prompt medical evaluation.

Foamy Urine: Excessive foaming or bubbly urine may indicate the presence of excess protein in the urine, which can be a sign of kidney damage or disease.

High Blood Pressure

Kidney disease can contribute to high blood pressure, and uncontrolled hypertension can further damage the kidneys. Seek medical attention if:

Blood Pressure Readings: Your blood pressure consistently measures higher than normal (above 140/90 mmHg), even after making lifestyle changes or using prescribed medications.

Uncontrolled Hypertension: Despite medication and lifestyle changes, if your blood pressure remains high or fluctuates significantly, consult with your healthcare provider for further evaluation and management.

Unexplained Weight Gain

Sudden or unexplained weight gain, especially if it is accompanied by swelling, may indicate fluid retention due to kidney dysfunction. Seek medical advice if:

Rapid Weight Gain: Significant weight gain over a short period, particularly if it is associated with swelling or discomfort, may require medical evaluation to determine the underlying cause.

Persistent Pain

Pain or discomfort in the lower back, sides, or abdomen that does not improve with natural remedies or lifestyle changes may need medical assessment. Common causes include:

Kidney Stones: Severe, persistent pain in the back or side may indicate kidney stones, which require medical treatment if they cause significant discomfort or complications.
Infections: Pain accompanied by fever or chills may signal a kidney infection (pyelonephritis) that requires antibiotics and medical intervention.

Sudden Changes in Health

Any sudden or severe changes in health should be evaluated promptly. These include:

Nausea and Vomiting: Persistent nausea or vomiting, especially if accompanied by a loss of appetite, can be a sign of worsening kidney function or complications.

Confusion or Difficulty Concentrating: Cognitive changes such as confusion, difficulty concentrating, or disorientation may indicate a buildup of toxins in the blood due to impaired kidney function.

Results from Routine Tests

Routine medical tests can provide important information about kidney health. Seek medical advice if:

Elevated Lab Results: Blood tests showing elevated levels of creatinine or blood urea nitrogen (BUN), or abnormal urinalysis results, indicate that kidney function may be compromised and require further investigation.

Imaging Findings: Abnormal results from kidney imaging studies, such as ultrasounds or CT scans, should be reviewed with a healthcare provider to determine the appropriate course of action.

Complications of Kidney Disease

Kidney disease can lead to various complications that require prompt medical attention, including:

Electrolyte Imbalances: Abnormal levels of potassium, calcium, or other electrolytes can cause serious health issues and may require medical intervention.

End-Stage Renal Disease (ESRD): If kidney function deteriorates to the point where the kidneys can no longer maintain essential bodily functions, treatments such as dialysis or kidney transplantation may be necessary.

Recognizing when to seek medical attention is crucial for managing kidney health and preventing complications. Persistent symptoms, changes in urine output, high blood pressure, unexplained weight gain, persistent pain, sudden changes in health, and abnormal test results are key indicators that warrant professional evaluation. Early intervention can help manage kidney disease effectively and improve overall outcomes. Always consult with a healthcare provider if you have concerns about your kidney health or experience any concerning symptoms.

CHAPTER 8

Myths and Facts About Kidney Health

Understanding the truth about kidney health is essential for effective management and prevention of kidney disease. This chapter dispels common myths and provides factual information to help you make informed decisions about your kidney health.

Myth 1: Only People with High Blood Pressure or Diabetes Need to Worry About Their Kidneys

Fact: While high blood pressure and diabetes are significant risk factors for kidney disease, anyone can develop kidney issues. Factors such as genetic predisposition, lifestyle choices, and age also play a role. Regular kidney health check-ups are important for everyone, especially if you have risk factors or symptoms.

Myth 2: You Can't Improve Kidney Function Once It's Declined

Fact: While advanced kidney disease may not be reversible, early-stage kidney disease can often be managed and improved with lifestyle changes, dietary modifications, and appropriate medical treatment. Adopting a kidney-friendly lifestyle and managing underlying conditions can slow progression and improve kidney function.

Myth 3: Kidney Disease Always Causes Noticeable Symptoms

Fact: Kidney disease can be asymptomatic, especially in its early stages. Many people with kidney disease may not experience symptoms until the condition is quite advanced. Regular screenings and tests are crucial for early detection and management.

Myth 4: Herbal Supplements Are Safe for Kidney Health
Fact: While some herbal supplements may offer benefits for kidney health, others can be harmful, especially if taken in excess or without medical supervision. Certain herbs can interact with medications or exacerbate kidney issues. Always consult a healthcare provider before starting any new supplements.

Myth 5: Drinking Excessive Water Cures Kidney Problems
Fact: While staying hydrated is important for kidney health, drinking excessive amounts of water does not cure kidney problems and can even be harmful in certain situations, such as in advanced kidney disease where fluid intake needs to be monitored. Proper hydration should be balanced with medical advice tailored to individual health needs.

Myth 6: Eating Too Much Protein Causes Kidney Disease
Fact: While excessive protein intake can put extra strain on the kidneys, particularly in individuals with

pre-existing kidney conditions, a balanced diet with moderate protein is not a direct cause of kidney disease in healthy individuals. It's important to follow a diet that meets individual health needs and consult with a healthcare provider or dietitian.

Myth 7: Kidney Stones Are Always Caused by Dehydration
Fact: Dehydration can contribute to the formation of kidney stones, but other factors such as dietary habits, genetic predisposition, and underlying health conditions also play a role. Preventing kidney stones involves managing multiple risk factors, including adequate hydration, diet, and sometimes medication.

Myth 8: Kidney Health Is Not Affected by Emotional Well-being
Fact: Emotional well-being can impact kidney health. Chronic stress, anxiety, and depression can contribute to high blood pressure and other conditions that affect the kidneys. Managing stress through healthy coping mechanisms and seeking mental health support can benefit overall kidney health.

Myth 9: All Kidney Diseases Are Genetic
Fact: While genetic factors can contribute to certain kidney diseases, many kidney conditions are influenced by lifestyle factors, such as diet, exercise, and exposure to toxins. Preventative measures and

lifestyle changes can help reduce the risk of developing kidney disease, even if there is a genetic predisposition.

Myth 10: Kidney Health Only Matters for Older Adults
Fact: Kidney disease can affect individuals of all ages, including children and young adults. Risk factors like obesity, high blood pressure, diabetes, and a sedentary lifestyle can contribute to kidney issues at any age. Regular monitoring and proactive health management are important across the lifespan.

Myth 11: Once Kidney Disease Is Diagnosed, There's Nothing More You Can Do
Fact: Diagnosis of kidney disease is a starting point for management, not the end. With appropriate treatment, lifestyle modifications, and regular monitoring, many individuals with kidney disease can manage their condition effectively and maintain a good quality of life. Engaging in a comprehensive care plan can help slow disease progression and address symptoms.

Myth 12: Kidney Function Tests Are Only Needed for People with Kidney Disease
Fact: Kidney function tests, such as blood urea nitrogen (BUN) and creatinine levels, are important for everyone, particularly if you have risk factors for kidney disease. Regular testing can help detect

early signs of kidney dysfunction and guide timely intervention.

Understanding the facts about kidney health can help dispel myths and encourage proactive management and prevention. Regular check-ups, informed lifestyle choices, and effective management of risk factors are key to maintaining kidney health and preventing disease. Stay informed, consult with healthcare professionals, and make choices that support your overall well-being.

CHAPTER 9

Conclusion

Kidney health is a crucial aspect of overall well-being, and maintaining healthy kidneys requires a comprehensive approach that includes understanding the functions of the kidneys, recognizing common diseases, and implementing effective prevention and management strategies.

Key Takeaways:
Understanding Kidney Function: The kidneys play a vital role in filtering blood, maintaining fluid balance, and regulating electrolytes. Knowing how they function helps in recognizing the importance of their health.

Prevention and Management: Adopting a kidney-friendly diet, making lifestyle changes, and using natural remedies can significantly support kidney health and potentially slow the progression of kidney disease. However, these should complement, not replace, conventional medical treatments.

When to Seek Medical Attention: It is crucial to recognize the signs that indicate worsening kidney function or complications. Persistent symptoms, changes in urine output, and abnormal test results warrant prompt medical evaluation.

Debunking Myths: Dispelling myths about kidney health helps in making informed decisions. Understanding the facts, such as the role of hydration, the impact of dietary choices, and the need for regular monitoring, ensures better management and prevention.

Holistic Approach: Integrating natural remedies, lifestyle changes, and holistic therapies can complement conventional treatments and improve quality of life. However, any new approach should be discussed with healthcare providers to ensure it is safe and appropriate.

Ultimately, maintaining kidney health is a proactive endeavor that involves regular monitoring, informed lifestyle choices, and effective management of health conditions. By staying informed and working closely with healthcare professionals, you can enhance your kidney health and overall well-being, making informed decisions that support long-term health.

Your journey towards better kidney health is a combination of awareness, proactive measures, and medical guidance. Embrace a balanced approach, and take control of your health to ensure a brighter and healthier future.

Glossary of Terms

Acute Kidney Injury (AKI): A sudden and rapid decline in kidney function, often caused by illness, injury, or medication. It is usually reversible with prompt treatment.

Chronic Kidney Disease (CKD): A long-term, progressive decline in kidney function that can lead to end-stage renal disease. It is typically diagnosed based on decreased kidney function over several months or years.

Dialysis: A medical treatment that artificially removes waste products and excess fluids from the blood when the kidneys are no longer able to perform these functions adequately.

End-Stage Renal Disease (ESRD): The final stage of chronic kidney disease where kidney function is severely impaired, requiring dialysis or a kidney transplant to sustain life.

Estimated Glomerular Filtration Rate (eGFR): A measure of kidney function that estimates how well the kidneys are filtering waste from the blood. It is calculated using blood creatinine levels, age, sex, and other factors.

Herbal Remedy: A treatment using plants or plant extracts to support health or treat illness. Herbal remedies can include teas, tinctures, capsules, and topical applications.

Hypertension: High blood pressure, which can damage blood vessels in the kidneys over time and contribute to kidney disease.

Nephrologist: A medical specialist who focuses on the diagnosis and treatment of kidney diseases and conditions.

Proteinuria: The presence of excess protein in the urine, which can be an indicator of kidney damage or disease.

Uremia: A condition characterized by high levels of waste products in the blood due to severe kidney dysfunction, leading to symptoms such as fatigue, nausea, and confusion.

Supplement and Herbal Remedy Dosages

Note: Always consult a healthcare provider before starting any supplements or herbal remedies, especially if you have kidney disease or are taking other medications.

Omega-3 Fatty Acids: 1,000 to 3,000 mg daily. This dosage is typically divided into multiple doses and can be adjusted based on individual needs and health conditions.

Coenzyme Q10 (CoQ10): 100 to 300 mg daily. Start with a lower dose and increase as needed, based on your healthcare provider's recommendations.

Vitamin D: 600 to 2,000 IU daily, depending on blood levels and individual needs. Higher doses may be prescribed for those with severe deficiency, under medical supervision.

Probiotics: 1 to 10 billion CFUs (colony-forming units) daily. The specific strain and dosage may vary based on the health condition and probiotic product.

Dandelion Root: 1 to 2 grams of dried root, taken as a tea or capsule, up to three times daily.

Nettle Leaf: 300 to 600 mg of dried leaf extract daily, often divided into two or three doses.

Astragalus: 500 to 1,000 mg of root extract daily, typically divided into two doses.

Corn Silk: 1 to 2 cups of corn silk tea daily, or as directed by a healthcare provider.

Sample Kidney-Friendly Meal Plans

Note: These meal plans are general guidelines. Personal needs may vary, and it's essential to consult a dietitian or healthcare provider for individualized recommendations.

Day 1
Breakfast: Oatmeal with fresh blueberries, a small handful of walnuts, and a sprinkle of cinnamon.
Lunch: Grilled chicken breast with a side of quinoa and steamed broccoli.
Snack: Apple slices with a small serving of almond butter.
Dinner: Baked salmon with a lemon-dill glaze, served with roasted sweet potatoes and a mixed green salad with a light vinaigrette.

Day 2
Breakfast: Greek yogurt with strawberries and a tablespoon of chia seeds.
Lunch: Lentil soup with a side of whole-grain bread and a mixed vegetable salad.
Snack: A small serving of carrots and cucumber slices with hummus.
Dinner: Stir-fried tofu with bell peppers, snap peas, and brown rice.

Day 3
Breakfast: Smoothie made with spinach, banana, and almond milk, with a tablespoon of flaxseeds.
Lunch: Turkey and avocado wrap using a whole-grain tortilla, with a side of mixed greens.
Snack: A handful of unsalted pumpkin seeds.
Dinner: Grilled shrimp with a side of asparagus and a small portion of couscous.

Day 4

Breakfast: Scrambled eggs with spinach and tomatoes, served with a slice of whole-grain toast.
Lunch: Chickpea and vegetable salad with a lemon-tahini dressing.
Snack: A pear and a small handful of sunflower seeds.
Dinner: Baked chicken thighs with a side of sautéed kale and brown rice.

Day 5
Breakfast: Chia pudding made with almond milk and topped with sliced strawberries.
Lunch: Quinoa salad with cucumbers, cherry tomatoes, and a lemon-herb dressing.
Snack: A small serving of mixed berries.
Dinner: Stuffed bell peppers with ground turkey, brown rice, and a side of steamed green beans.
These sample meal plans focus on foods that are generally low in sodium, potassium, and phosphorus, which are important for kidney health. Adjustments may be needed based on individual dietary needs and kidney function.